Healthy Mom, Healthy Baby

DIABETES & PREGNANCY

A GUIDE TO YOUR ANTENATAL CARE DURING PREGNANCY

LATOYA EFEADUE

A Note to Readers

The information in this book is not intended or implied to be a substitute for professional medical advice, diagnosis or treatment. All content in these pages--including text, charts, illustrations, graphics, and photographs--is for general information purposes only.

You are encouraged to confirm any information obtained from or through this book with other sources and to review all information regarding any medical condition or treatment with your physician or healthcare professional.

Never disregard professional medical advice, forego or delay seeking medical treatment because of something you have read in this book.

ISBN-13: 978-1546793038
ISBN-10: 1546793038

Contributors

SHARMAINE SCOTT, MSN, RN
High-Risk OB Nurse Case Manager
Women & Infant Health Services Department
Grady Health System
Atlanta, GA

JOHNNIE HALL, BSN, RN
High-Risk OB Nurse Case Manager
Women & Infant Health Services Department
Grady Health System
Atlanta, GA

ERIN STEBER, MS, RD, LD
Registered Dietitian
Atlanta, GA

THE

Table of Contents

Chapter 1
Diabetes: Understanding the Basics

Chapter 2
Managing Your Diabetes

Chapter 3
Meal Planning

Chapter 4
Staying Healthy After Pregnancy

Appendix
Sample Menus

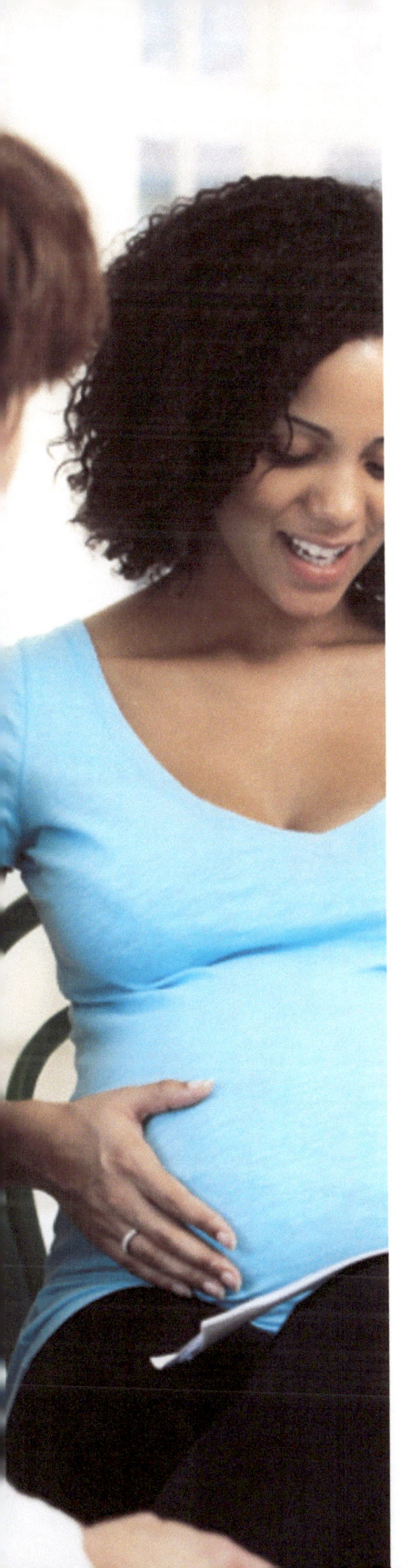

CHAPTER 1

DIABETES: UNDERSTANDING THE BASICS

Diabetes is the condition in which the body does not properly process food for use as energy. Most of the food we eat is turned into glucose, or sugar for our bodies to use for energy. The pancreas, an organ that lies near the stomach, makes a hormone called insulin to help glucose get into the cells of our bodies. When you have diabetes, your body either doesn't make enough insulin or cannot use its own insulin as well as it should. This causes sugars to build up in your blood. This is also why many people refer to diabetes as "sugar."

Diabetes can cause serious health complications including heart disease, blindness, kidney failure, and lower-extremity amputations. It is also the seventh leading cause of death in the United States.

Also, diabetes can be a hereditary condition, meaning, if you have a family history of this condition you are more likely to develop diabetes. It can be more common in certain ethnic groups such as those of Asian, African or Caribbean descent. Additionally, diabetes can be related to lifestyle choices such as poor eating habits and lack of exercise.

Take a look below to see how your body breaks down the food you eat.

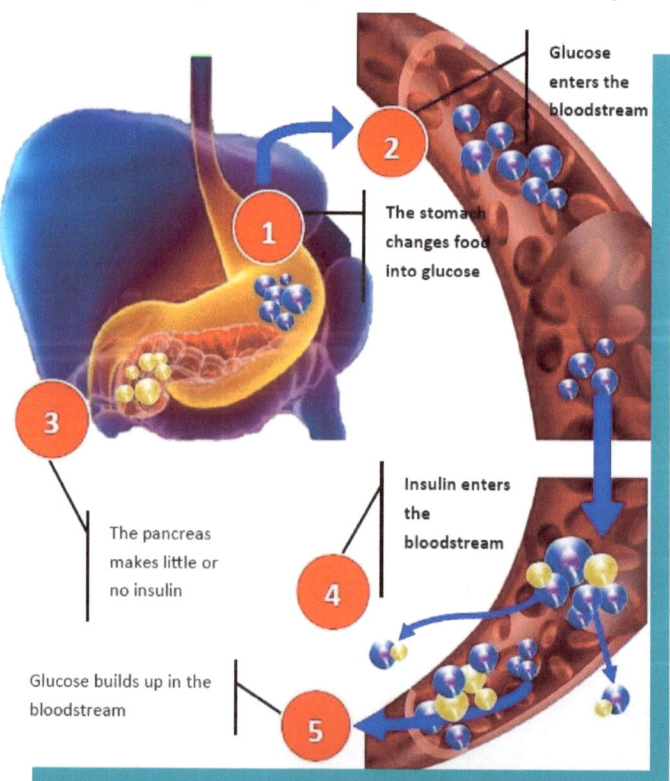

Types of Diabetes

People most commonly develop diabetes early in childhood, later in life after age 45, or during pregnancy. Pregnancy normally increases the body's need for insulin, therefore, most women are routinely tested during pregnancy between 24-28 weeks. There are three main types of diabetes: Type 1, Type 2 and Gestational Diabetes.

Type 1 Diabetes

Also called insulin-dependent diabetes, this type of diabetes most often occurs in children and young adults. People with Type 1 Diabetes produce little or no insulin and must follow a meal plan, exercise plan, and take insulin.

Type 2 Diabetes

Also called non-insulin-dependent diabetes, Type 2 Diabetes is more common and usually occurs in adults. Blood glucose in people with Type 2 diabetes can be controlled by a meal plan, exercise plan, oral medication, insulin, or a combination of all four.

Gestational Diabetes (GDM)

Gestational diabetes mellitus (GDM) develops during pregnancy and usually goes away once the baby is born. GDM develops in about 2-5% of all pregnancies and if not treated can cause health problems for mother and fetus.

Gestational Diabetes

Gestational diabetes (pronounced jess-TAY-shun-ul die-uh-BEET-eez) is one of the most common health problems for pregnant women. About 6-7 percent of pregnancies are complicated by diabetes mellitus (DM) and 90 percent of these cases are women with gestational diabetes mellitus (GDM).

When you have diabetes, your body cannot use the sugars and starches (carbohydrates) it takes in as food to make energy. As a result, your body collects extra sugar in your blood.

If not treated, gestational diabetes can cause health problems for mother and fetus. The good news is that gestational diabetes can be treated, especially if it's found early in the pregnancy. There are some things that women with gestational diabetes can do to keep themselves well and their pregnancies healthy.

Controlling gestational diabetes is the key to a healthy pregnancy. This booklet gives women who have been diagnosed with this condition the information they need to talk to health care providers, dietitians, family members and friends about gestational diabetes.

Who's at Risk for Diabetes

Numerous factors raise a pregnant woman's risk of developing gestational diabetes. Some but not all women with gestational diabetes are overweight before getting pregnant or have diabetes in the family. It is more common in Native American, Alaskan Native, Hispanic, Asian and Black women, however, it can also be found in White women too.

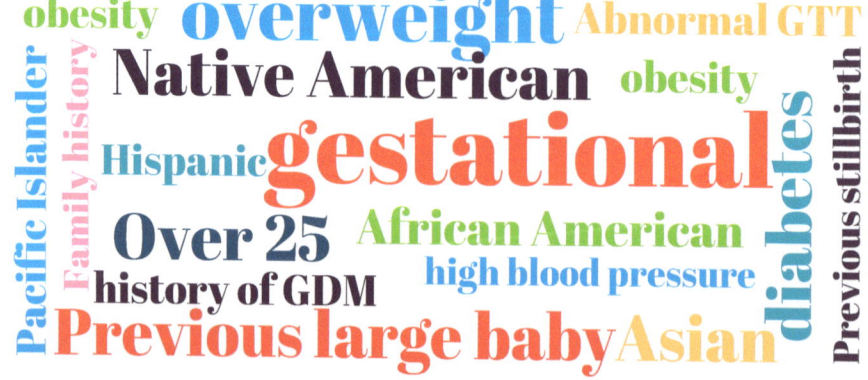

What Are The Symptoms

Most women with gestational diabetes have no symptoms, though a few may experience any of the symptoms listed below:

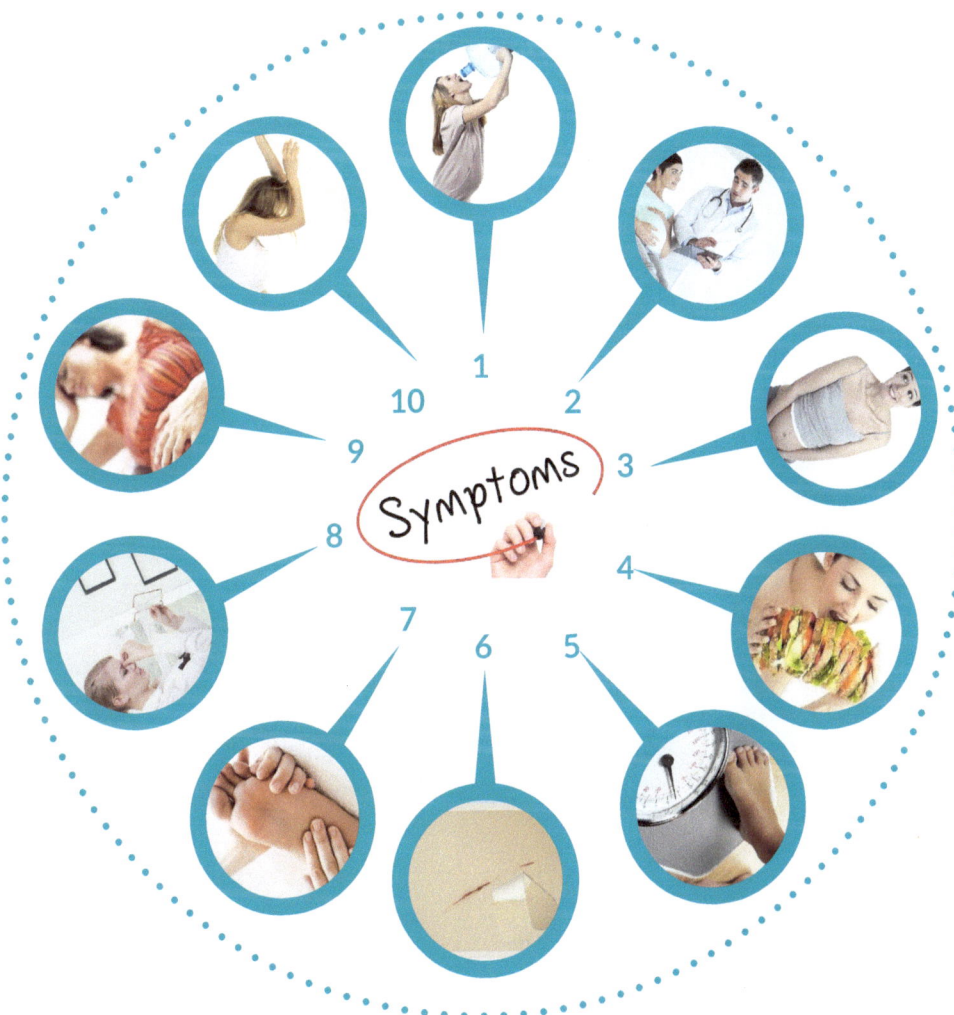

Answer Key

1. Extreme thirst 2. Frequent Infections 3. Excessive urination 4. Extreme hunger 5. Sudden weight loss 6. Slow healing cuts or sores 7. Numbness or tingling in hands/feet 8. Changes in eye sight 9. Tiredness 10. Lack of energy

How is Diabetes Diagnosed

Gestational diabetes is commonly diagnosed during the routine testing that occurs as part of your medical care during pregnancy. In a normal pregnancy, blood sugars are about 20% lower than women who aren't pregnant because the developing fetus absorbs some of the glucose from the mother's blood. Diabetes is evident if blood sugar levels are higher than expected for pregnancy. In order to find gestational diabetes in its earliest form, the provider performs an oral glucose tolerance test which includes drinking a heavily sugared drink before testing the blood so that the body's sugar-processing ability is maximally challenged.

Women who are overweight or have any risk factors such as; family history of diabetes, gestational diabetes in a previous pregnancy or symptoms suggesting diabetes, she will undergo testing at the first prenatal visit. After 24 weeks of gestation, all others complete the glucose tolerance test for diabetes, most often between 24 and 28 weeks.

Screening

A screening test can only provide your risk, or probability that a particular condition exists. When the results of a screening test are positive, diagnostic tests can provide a definitive answer.

Take a look at the following flow chart to review the screening process for gestational diabetes.

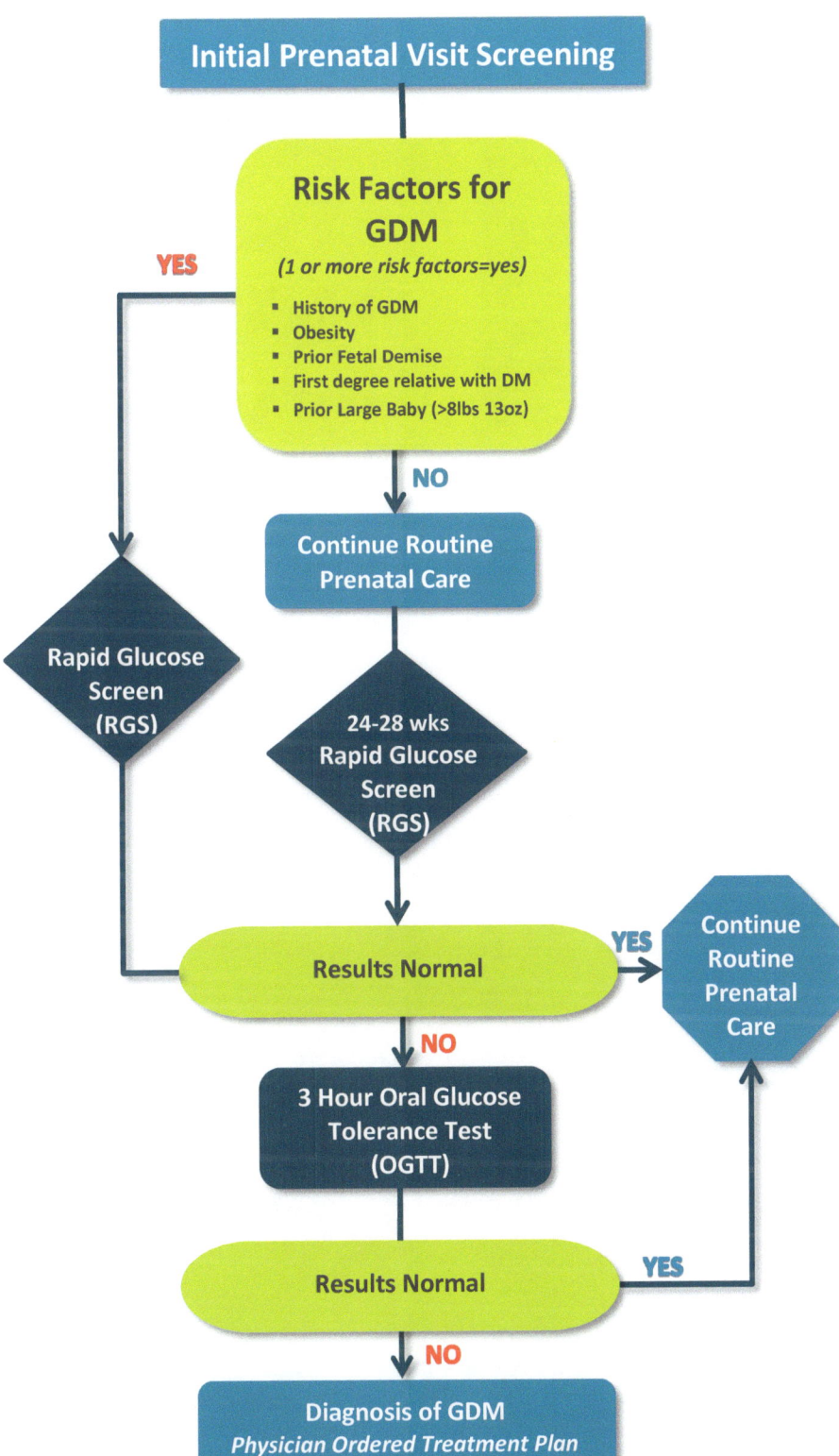

Initial Prenatal Visit Screening

Risk Factors for GDM
(1 or more risk factors=yes)

- History of GDM
- Obesity
- Prior Fetal Demise
- First degree relative with DM
- Prior Large Baby (>8lbs 13oz)

YES

NO

Continue Routine Prenatal Care

Rapid Glucose Screen (RGS)

24-28 wks Rapid Glucose Screen (RGS)

Results Normal

YES

Continue Routine Prenatal Care

NO

3 Hour Oral Glucose Tolerance Test (OGTT)

Results Normal

YES

NO

Diagnosis of GDM
Physician Ordered Treatment Plan

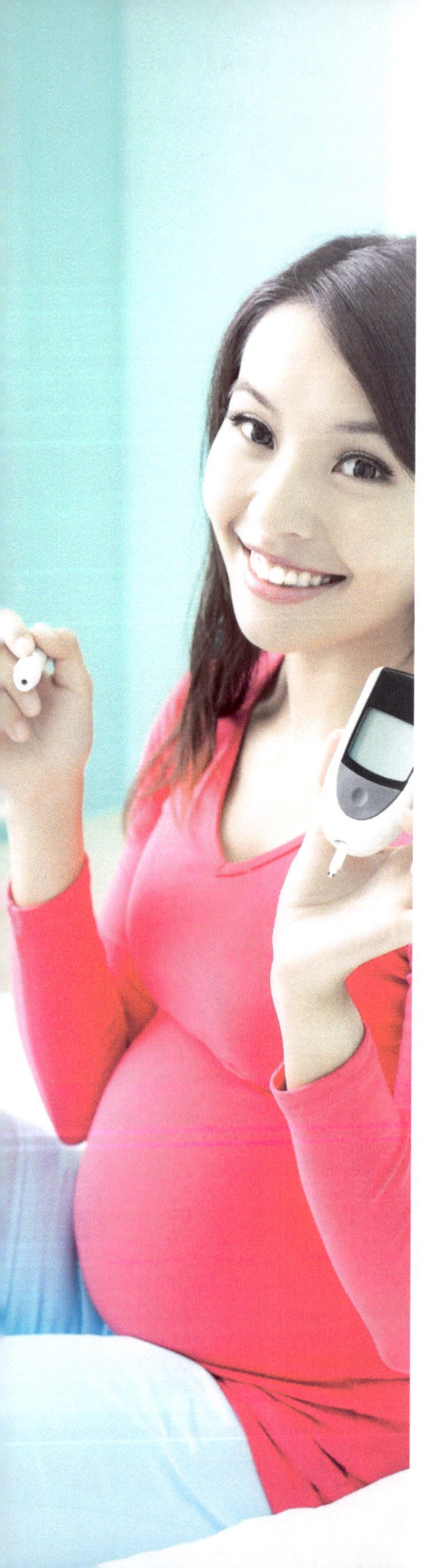

CHAPTER 2

MANAGING
YOUR DIABETES

Over 130 million women give birth each year and for women with Gestational diabetes, while the risks and challenges are of course magnified, the reality is that you can successfully navigate the before and after phases of pregnancy. Although gestational diabetes usually does not cause birth defects or deformities, it is important for you to manage your diabetes and maintain a healthy lifestyle through eating healthy foods and regular exercise to prevent further complications. Most developmental or physical defects happen during the first trimester of pregnancy, between the 1st and 8th week, while gestational diabetes typically develops around or after the 24th week of pregnancy. Women with gestational diabetes usually have normal blood sugar levels during the first trimester, allowing the body and body systems of the fetus to develop normally.

Although you have gestational diabetes, it will not cause diabetes in your baby, however, your baby is at higher risk for developing type 2 diabetes later in life. As your child grows, things, like eating a healthy diet, maintaining a healthy weight, and getting regular, moderate physical activity, may help to reduce that risk. If your baby was macrosomic, or large bodied at birth, then he or she is at a higher risk for childhood and adult obesity. Large babies are also at greater risk for getting type 2 diabetes and often are diagnosed at an earlier age *(younger than 30)* than those who were small bodied babies.

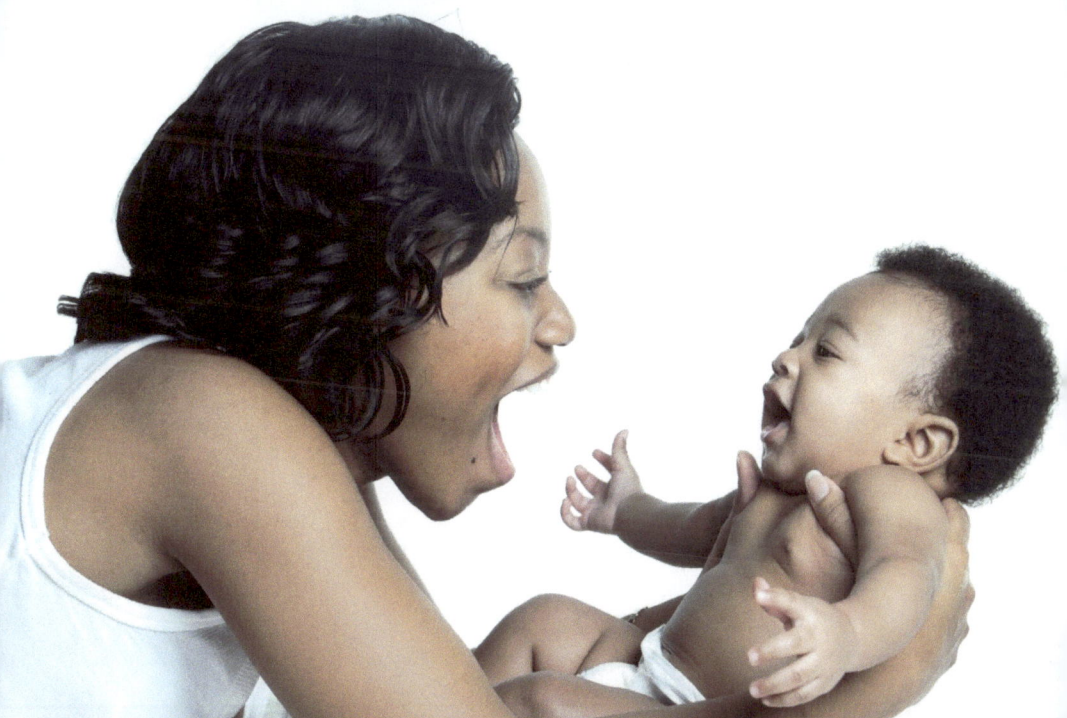

Gestational Diabetes & My Baby

Most women with gestational diabetes have healthy pregnancies and healthy babies. Getting good treatment makes all the difference. However, gestational diabetes that's not carefully managed can lead to uncontrolled blood sugar levels and cause problems for you and your baby, including an increased likelihood of needing a C-section to deliver. Also, untreated gestational diabetes can result in a baby's death either before or shortly after birth. For the health of you and your baby, it is important to do the following:

- Maintain a healthy blood sugar level
- Eat a healthy diet
- Get regular, moderate physical activity
- Maintain a healthy weight

During pregnancy, the glucose, also known as sugar from foods that you eat cross through the placenta to give the baby energy. As a result of gestational diabetes, the baby receives more glucose than is needed and the baby then stores it as fat.

If your blood glucose levels are uncontrolled, your baby may be likely to have certain complications like:

- Injuries during delivery because of their size
- Low blood sugar when they're born
- Jaundice, a treatable condition that makes the skin yellowish
- Pre-term birth
- Temporary breathing problems

COMMON COMPLICATIONS

Macrosomia *(Large Baby)* (pronounced mak-ros-SOSHM-ee-uh)
Newborn who's significantly larger than average and weighs more than 8 pounds, 13 ounces (4,000 grams), regardless of his or her gestational age. Fetal macrosomia may complicate vaginal delivery and could put the baby at risk of injury during birth. Fetal macrosomia also puts the baby at increased risk of health problems after birth. The most common complication is shoulder dystocia.

Hypoglycemia (pronounced high-po-gl-eye-SEEM-ee-uh)
Newborn's blood sugar is too low. You may need to start breastfeeding right away to get more glucose into the baby's system. If it's not possible for you to start feedings, the baby may need to get glucose through a thin, plastic tube in their arm that puts glucose directly into the blood.

Jaundice (pronounced JAWN-diss)
Newborn jaundice is a yellow discoloration in a newborn baby's skin and eyes. Infant jaundice occurs because the baby's blood contains an excess of bilirubin (bil-ih-ROO-bin), a yellow-colored pigment of red blood cells. Treatment of infant jaundice often isn't necessary, and most cases that need treatment respond well to noninvasive therapy.

Respiratory Distress Syndrome (RDS)
The newborn has trouble breathing. The baby might need oxygen or other help breathing if they have RDS. It is commonly associated with cesarean sections, prematurity and delayed lung maturity.

Exercise, Stress & Medications

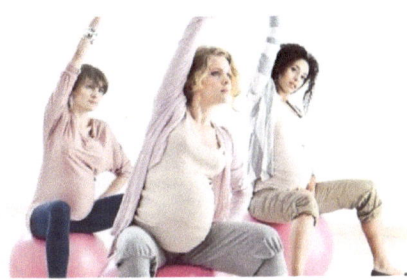

Exercise is an important part of pregnancy. It can help to prevent back pain and increase strength and endurance. For women with gestational diabetes, exercise is also a good way to improve your body's own insulin production and lower your blood glucose. Additionally, exercise can also prevent you from needing to take medication such as insulin to lower your blood glucose. A normal 20 to 30-minute walk, especially after eating, is a great way to keep your blood glucose in a normal range. Always check with your doctor before starting an exercise program. If you are exercising and feel any excessive cramping, pressure, or start to feel bad in general, stop exercising immediately.

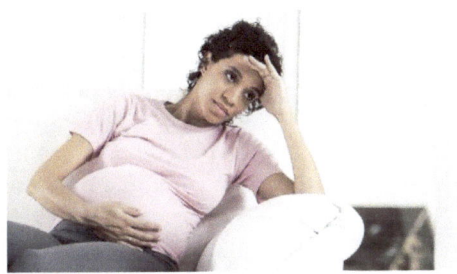

Pregnancy, even under normal conditions, is stressful and added stress can cause your blood glucose levels to be higher than normal. So when you have gestational diabetes, managing and lowering your stress level is of great importance because of how it can affect blood glucose.

Here are some ways to lower your stress level.

- Get enough sleep each day or take naps if you are tired
- Develop a daily routine
- Exercise or go for a walk
- Find quiet time for yourself to do something you enjoy like reading or listening to music
- Practice relaxation techniques such as deep breathing exercises or guided imagery

Medication may be prescribed when diet alone is not enough. In many cases, the meal plan will work to control your blood glucose. If medication is prescribed, it is not a replacement for the meal plan. You must still follow the meal plan. If you were on medication for diabetes before your pregnancy, you may need more medication during your pregnancy. Your provider will decide what medication will work best for you and the healthcare team will educate you on how to take your medication.

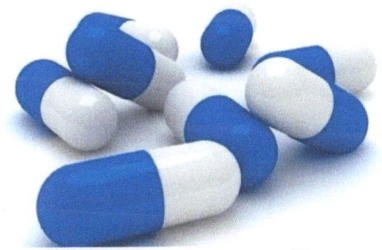

Blood Glucose Monitoring

There are 2 steps in the first phase of treatment of gestational diabetes, which include the following:

1. Checking your glucose
    -   Checking your glucose will become a part of your daily routine and your glucometer will give you immediate results.
2. Maintaining target glucose levels
    -   It is important for you to record and use your glucose history as a guide to work with your provider and healthcare team to determine what your target goals should be and to develop a program of regular blood glucose monitoring to manage your condition.

When should I take my blood glucose?

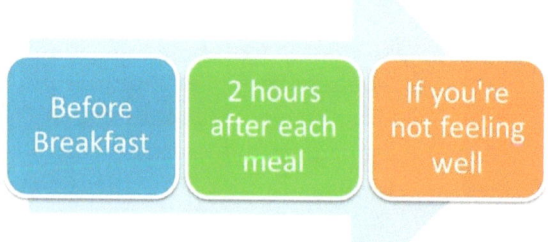

You will be required to monitor your blood glucose levels by pricking your finger about 3-4 times each day, before and after meals, if you're not feeling well or as instructed by your provider.

How to keep my blood glucose under control

Even though your glucose level changes during the day, there is a healthy range for these levels and your goal is to keep your glucose level within theses ranges. The following chart outlines the healthy target range for each time you test.

HEALTHY TARGET RANGE FOR GLUCOSE LEVELS	
Time of Blood Sugar Test	**Healthy Target Levels** *(mg/dl)*
Fasting Glucose Level	Less than or equal to 95
One hour after eating	Less than or equal to 140
Two hours after eating	Less than or equal to 120

If your blood glucose is lower than 60 or higher than 180, write down a diary of your activities and meals that might help explain why your blood glucose is not in the healthy target range. Also, talk to your healthcare provider about what to do if your glucose level is outside the healthy target listed in this book. You may have to adjust your treatment plan to get your levels back in range.

Your healthcare provider will show you how to test your glucose level and will give you detailed information about glucose testing. The following steps are only meant to give you a basic idea of what is involved in testing:

How to Check Your Blood Glucose

Gather all of your supplies and wash your hands with warm water and soap.

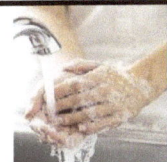

Insert test strip. Meter automatically turns on.

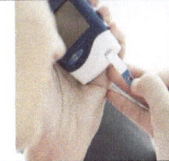

Prick your finger with a small needle called a lancet (pronounced LAN-sett). Always stick the side of your finger. Squeeze out a drop of blood. (Note: If you cleaned your finger with an alcohol swab, make sure that your finger has dried or wipe the first drop of blood away).

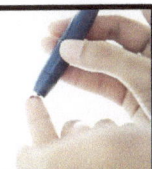

Apply the blood to the test strip. Touch and hold the blood drop to the edge of the strip and make sure it fills the window of the strip completely.

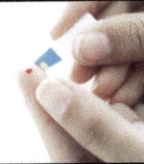

Read results. Record results in your blood glucose diary.

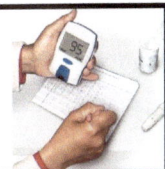

Signs & Symptoms

Low and high blood glucose have similar symptoms. Therefore, it is important for you to manage your glucose appropriately and always check your blood glucose when you're not feeling well. The table below gives you common symptoms, causes and tells you how each should be managed. If you're uncertain, always notify your healthcare provider.

Low Blood Glucose

If your blood glucose level drops below 60 mg/dL at any time, you have hypoglycemia (hypo means low, and glycemia means sugar). Low blood sugar can be dangerous. Hypoglycemia is not common in women with gestational diabetes, but you are at greater risk for it if you take insulin. The table shown here describes some reasons that low blood sugar might occur and some of its symptoms.

KNOW THE SYMPTOMS OF LOW BLOOD SUGAR	
Why does low blood sugar occur?	How might I feel if have low blood sugar
• Too much exercise • Skipping meals or snacks • Delaying meals or snacks • Not eating often enough • Too much insulin	• Very hungry • Very tired • Shaky or trembling • Sweating or clamminess • Nervous • Confused • Like you're going to pass out or faint • Blurred vision Or…You might feel fine

What to do

HOW TO MANAGE SYMPTOMS OF LOW BLOOD SUGAR	
Blood glucose is lower than 60 mg/dL AND you are having any of the above symptoms:	Eat your scheduled snack or meal and remember to stay on your planned meal schedule.
If it is during the night and you are having any of the above symptoms :	Have ½ cup milk and 4 crackers with peanut butter or cheese.

High Blood Glucose

If your blood glucose level is above 130 mg/dL at any time, you have hyperglycemia (hyper means high, and glycemia means sugar). High blood sugar can also be dangerous. The table shown here describes some reasons that high blood sugar might occur and some of its symptoms.

KNOW THE SYMPTOMS OF HIGH BLOOD SUGAR	
Why does high blood sugar occur?	**Why does high blood sugar occur?**
• Too much food • Infection, fever or illness • Emotional stress • Not enough medication	• Drowsiness • Very tired • Blurry vision • Sweating or clamminess • Increased thirst • Confused • Loss of appetite, nausea or vomiting • Increased urination • Weakness or aching all over Or...You might feel fine

What to do

HOW TO MANAGE SYMPTOMS OF HIGH BLOOD SUGAR	
Blood glucose is higher than the normal range BUT less than 160 mg/dL:	Take a walk and drink water
Blood glucose is higher than 160 twice in one day and you have any of the above symptoms.	Call your provider or Nurse

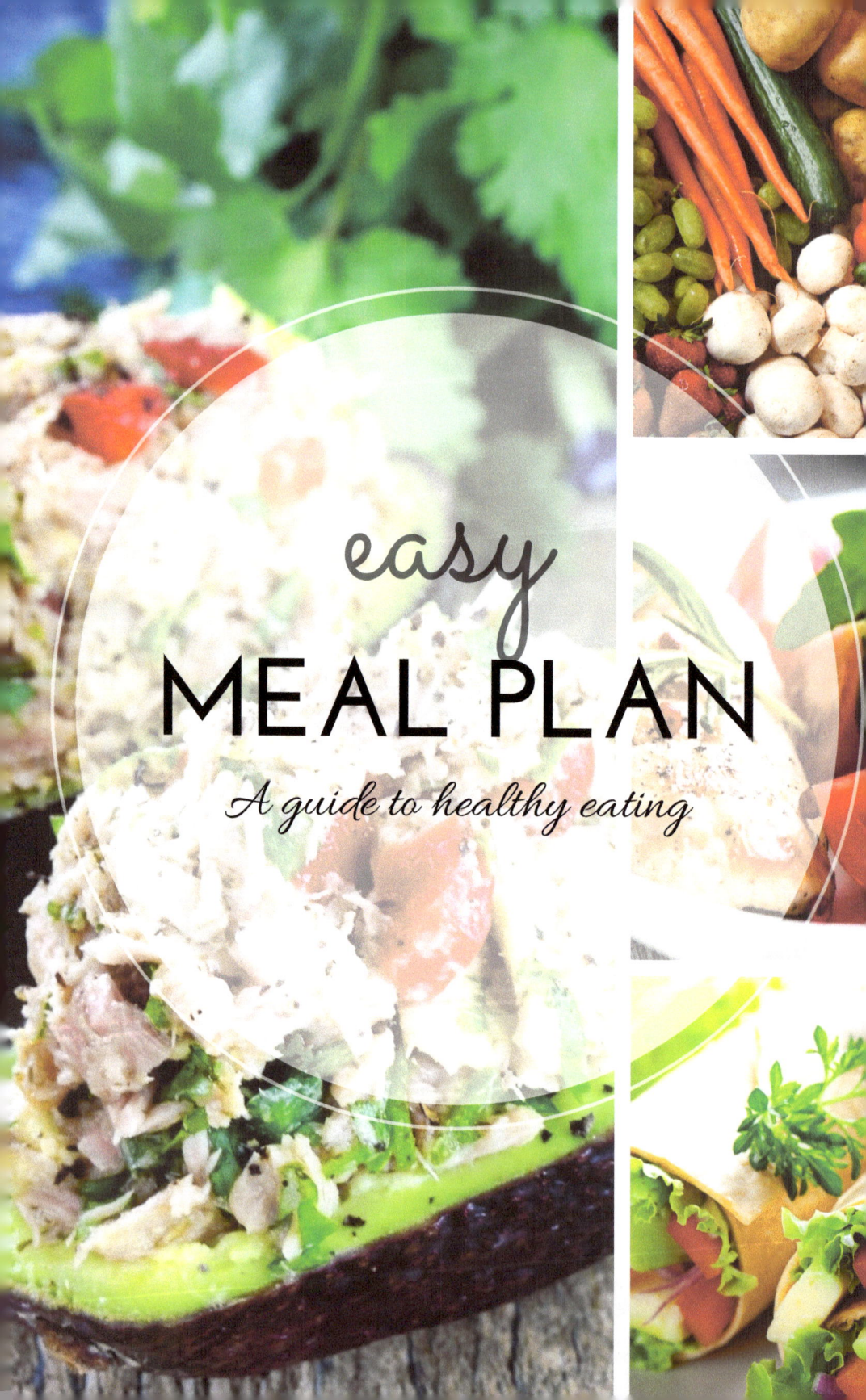

easy
MEAL PLAN

A guide to healthy eating

For anyone with diabetes, meal planning is important for controlling blood glucose. Different foods can increase your blood glucose levels more than others. The goal of a meal plan is to keep your blood glucose in a normal and consistent range for the entire day. By measuring the foods you eat, especially foods that contain carbohydrates, you can achieve this goal.

A healthy diet is one that includes a balance of foods from all the food groups, giving you the nutrients, vitamins, and minerals needed for a healthy pregnancy. For women with gestational diabetes, a balanced diet also helps to keep blood sugar levels in the healthy target range.

The information in this booklet is specific to women who have been diagnosed with gestational diabetes. These guidelines are not appropriate for all pregnant women, nor do they apply to women who are not pregnant or who have other types of diabetes. It is important that you follow the plan as outlined by your health care provider.

Your Meal Plan

It is important that you eat a total of six times per day to keep your blood glucose in a normal range throughout the day. Your daily meals should consist of three meals and three snacks per day. It is also recommended that you eat every 2 ½ to 3 hours.

Your meal plan should be divided into 6 categories:

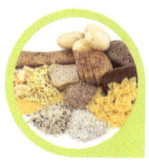 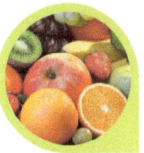 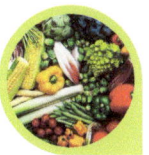 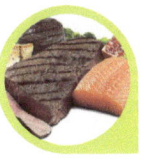 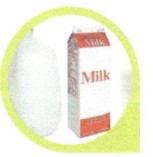 

BREADS & STARCHES	FRUITS	VEGETABLES	PROTEINS	MILK	FATS

You will not need to count calories, but you will have to count the number of servings of food that you eat from each food group. The amount of food in a serving depends on the type of food. For example, one slice of bread equals one serving, and a half bagel also equals one serving, where as a whole bagel equals two servings.

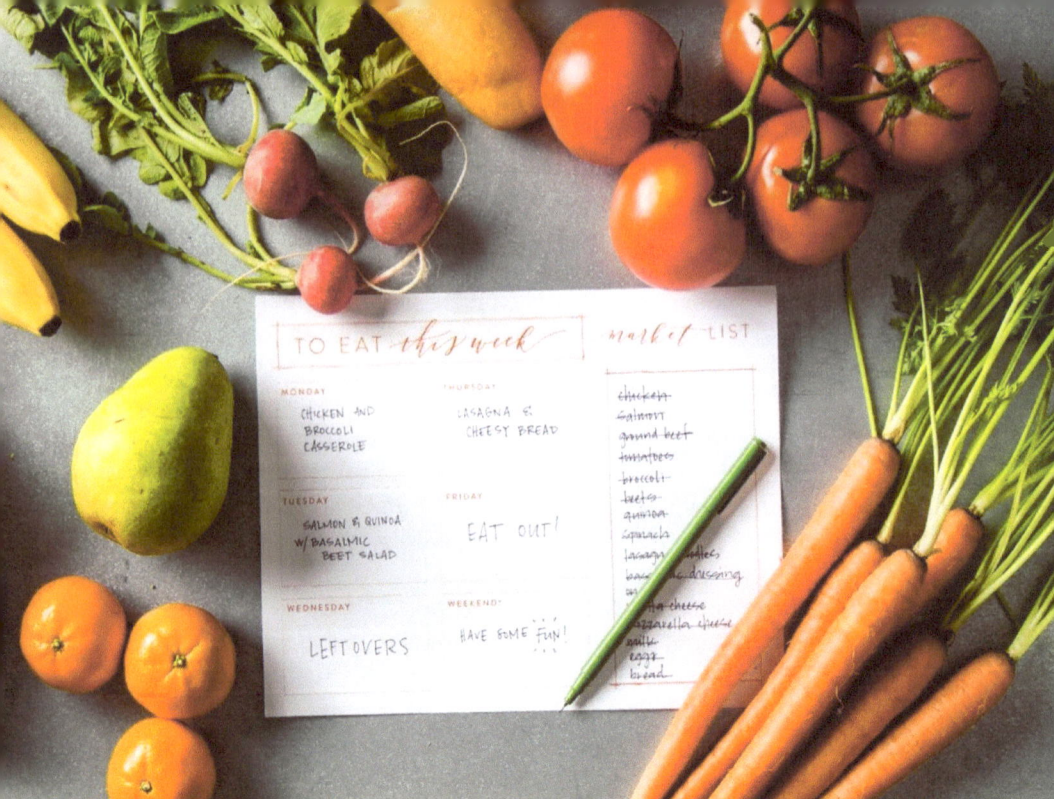

Planning Your Meals

When planning your meals it is very important to follow these steps:

- Follow your meal plan closely. Eat your meals and snacks at the same time each day.
- Try to eat all the food on your meal plan. If you are not able to finish or you are not hungry, choose to eat the foods from the carbohydrate groups, especially if you are taking prescribed medications for your diabetes.
- Take your blood glucose machine, test strips, and blood glucose diary wherever you go.
- If you plan to travel and you are away from home, take your own food or take money to buy food.
- Write your blood glucose results in your diary as soon as you take it. If your blood glucose is high, write down what you ate and drank for the two hours before, so that your healthcare team can help make any needed changes in your meal plan.

Carbohydrates

Carbohydrates are often at the center of a healthy diet for a woman with gestational diabetes.

Carbohydrates are nutrients that come from certain foods, like grain products, fruits, and vegetables. During digestion, your body breaks down most carbohydrates into simple sugars, like glucose, which is your body's main source of energy.

Eating carbohydrates can also have an affect on your blood sugar level. For instance, if you eat a few carbohydrates at a meal, your blood sugar level goes up a small amount. If you eat a lot of carbohydrates at a meal, your blood sugar level goes up a large amount.

The Carbohydrate Category

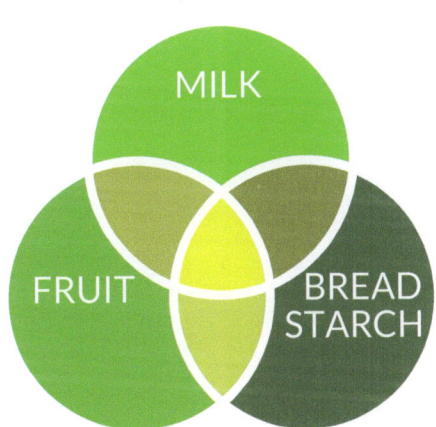

Things to Know About Carbohydrates

There are a few things you should know about carbohydrates and your healthy diet:

- You and your healthcare provider will come up with a healthy diet for you that includes the proper amount of carbohydrates to maintain a healthy pregnancy.
- Not getting enough carbohydrates can also cause problems. So, you should only limit your carbohydrate intake if advised to do so by your health care provider.

- Some women with gestational diabetes may need to avoid high sugar foods, like sweets and desserts to keep their carbohydrate levels in line. But, even though these foods have more carbohydrates and sugars in each serving than other foods do, they can still be worked into a plan for healthy eating in most cases.

Reading A Food Label

It is very important to make sure that serving sizes of carbohydrate foods are measured. Often this means that you will need to read food labels to determine how much to eat.

Remember 1 serving of Carbohydrate = 15 grams of Carbohydrate

Take a look at this sample food label.

SAMPLE LABEL

READING THE LABEL

Nutrition Facts		
Serving Size: 1 cup		
Servings Per Container: 2		
Amount Per Serving		
Calories 260 Calories from Fat 120		
		% Daily Value
Total Fat	13g	20%
Saturated Fat	5g	25%
Cholesterol	30mg	10%
Sodium	660mg	28%
Total Carbohydrate	30mg	10%
Dietary Fiber	0g	0%
Sugar	5g	
Protein	5g	

How much can I have?

A serving is not always the whole container or package of food.

1 serving = 15 gm of Carbohydrates

When reading the label, look at the total amount carbohydrates *per serving.*

Example
1 Serving = 1 cup
Total Carbohydrates per serving = 30 gm
    1 serving of Carbohydrates = ½ cup
        This whole container = 2 cups

If You Ate
- Half of the container
    ⇒ 1 cup = 2 servings of Carbohydrates
- All of the container
    ⇒ 2 cups = 4 servings of Carbohydrates

The Milk Group

The Milk Group contains different types of milk and milk products. All milk and milk products contain sugar, so it is important to measure and count servings. On the diabetic meal plan, cheese is not in the milk group but in the Meat or Fat group.   The tables below shows how many cups of each type of milk group is equal to 1 carbohydrate serving.

THE MILK GROUP			
MILK		**LACTOSE INTOLERANCE OPTIONS**	
TYPE	SERVING SIZE	TYPE	SERVING SIZE
Skim	1 cup	Lactose free milk	1 cup
½ %	1 cup	Oat milk	1 cup
1 %	1 cup	Rice milk	1 cup
2 %	1 cup	Soy milk-*plain*	1 cup
Whole	1 cup	**YOGURT/PUDDING**	
Low-Fat Buttermilk	1 cup	Cottage Cheese	2 cups
Canned Skim Milk	½ cup	Fruit Yogurt *(light)*	1 cup
Evaporated Whole Milk	½ cup	Kefir	1 cup
Dry non-fat milk	⅓ cup	Yogurt *(Vanilla or Plain)*	1 cup
Goat milk	1 cup		

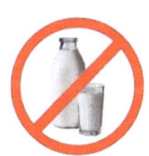

Milk Products to Avoid

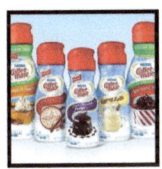

Coffee Creamers
Coffee-mate, Cremora, or Flavored Creams

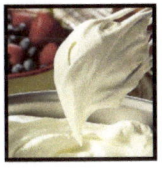

Creams
Light or heavy whipping cream

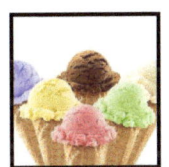

Others
Frappuccino's, Lattes, Ice Cream, Frozen Yogurt

The Fruit Group

Foods in the Fruit Group are naturally high in sugar and should be measured carefully. A serving of fresh fruit is a piece of fruit that you can hold in the palm of your hand. The following table shows food in each fruit group and the suggested portion size.

THE FRUIT GROUP			
FRESH, FROZEN OR UNSWEETENED CANNED FRUIT			
TYPE	**SERVING SIZE**	**TYPE**	**SERVING SIZE**
Apple (any kind)	1 small	Kiwi	1
Applesauce	½ cup	Mango	1 small
Apricots	4 medium	Nectarine	1
Apricots (canned)	½ cup	Orange	1 small
Banana	2 inch piece	Papaya	1 cup
Blackberries	¾ cup	Peach	1
Blueberries	¾ cup	Peach (canned)	½ cup
Cantaloupe	⅓ canteloupe	Pear	1 small
Cherries	12 cherries	Pear (canned)	½ cup
Cherries (canned)	½ cup	Pineapple	¾ cup
Figs	2	Pineapple (canned)	½ cup
Fruit Cocktail	½ cup	Plum	2
Grapefruit	½ grapefruit	Raspberries	1 cup
Grapes	15 small, 10 large	Strawberries	1 ¼ cup
Honeydew Melon	⅛ melon	Tangerine	2
DRIED FRUIT		**FRUIT JUICE**	
Apples	4 rings	Apple	½ cup
Apricot	7 halves	Cranberry	⅓ cup
Banana chips	¼ cup	Grape	⅓ cup
Cranberries	2 Tablespoons	Grapefruit	⅔ cup
Dates	2 ½ medium	Orange	½ cup
Prunes	3 medium	Pineapple	½ cup
Rasins	2 Tablespoons	Prune Juice	⅓ cup

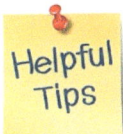

- Do NOT eat fruit with breakfast. This will cause your blood glucose to be high.
- Avoid canned fruit, unless packed in its own juice. Fresh or frozen fruit is always best.

- Avoid juices and consider having fresh fruit. Juices contain large amounts of sugar, so servings should be small.
- Dried fruits have had the water removed making the portion size smaller than fresh fruit.

The Bread & Starch Group

There is no end in sight to the debate as to whether grains help you lose weight, or if they promote weight gain. Even more importantly, do they help or hinder blood glucose, the main sugar found in the blood and the body's main source of energy? One thing is for sure. if you are going to eat grain foods, pick the ones that are the most nutritious. Choose whole grains. Whole grains are rich in vitamins, minerals, phytochemicals and fiber. Examples of grains include but are not limited to, wheat, rice, oats, cornmeal, and barley. Foods made from grains and some types of vegetables are called starches, which also provide carbohydrates which give our body energy. Bread, pasta, oatmeal, cereal, tortillas, and grits, which are made from these grains, are examples of starches. These foods can also be high in fiber, which takes longer to digest and therefore affect your blood glucose more slowly (i.e. whole wheat bread, prunes and other vegetables).

Reading labels is essential for this food group to make sure you are making the best choices. Every time you choose toeat a starchy food, make it count! Leave the processed white flour-based products, especially the ones with added sugar. The following table shows foods in each group and the suggested portion size.

THE BREAD & STARCH GROUP

BREADS		CEREAL	
TYPE	SERVING SIZE	TYPE	SERVING SIZE
Bagel	½ bagel	**BOXED OR DRY CEREALS**	
Bread stick (4 inch)	2 bread sticks	Bran cereal	½ cup
Bun (hamburger)	½ bun	Cereal with dried fruit	¼ cup
Bun (hot dog)	½ bun	Grape-nuts	¼ cup
English Muffin	½ muffin	Shredded wheat	½ cup
Pita (6 inch)	½ pita	Unsweetened (no fruit)	¾ cup
Raisin (unfrosted)	½ slice	**CEREAL COOKED WITH WATER**	
Reduced Calorie	2 slices	Cream of wheat	½ cup or ½ packet
Roll (small)	1 roll	Grits	½ cup or ½ packet
Rye or pumpernickel	1 slice	Oatmeal	½ cup or ½ packet
Tortilla (6 inch taco size)	1 tortilla	**GRAINS OR PASTAS**	
Wheat	1 slice	Cornmeal (dry)	3 tablespoons
White	1 slice	Couscous	⅓ cup
BREADS MADE WITH FAT		Flour (dry)	3 tablespoons
Biscuit (2 ½ inch)	1	Kasha	½ cup
Cheese with peanut butter	3	Oats	½ cup
Chow mein noodles	½ cup	Pasta or noodles	½ cup
Cornbread (2 inch cube)	1	Rice (cooked)	½ cup
Crackers	6 crackers	Risotto	½ cup
Crackers (round)	6	Wheat germ	½ cup
Croutons	1 cup	**STARCHY VEGETABLES**	
French fries	Small (16-25)	Beans (baked)	¼ cup
Muffin (small, no fruit)	1	Beans (dried)	½ cup cooked
Pancake (4 inch)	2	Beans (lima)	½ cup
Stuffing or dressing	½ cup	Corn	½ cup
Taco shell	1 shell	Corn on the cob	1 ear
CRACKERS & SNACKS		Lentils	½ cup cooked
Animal	8 crackers	Miso	3 tablespoons
Cheez-Its	22 crackers	Mixed vegetables	1 cup
Graham	3 squares	Peas	½ cup
Oyster	24 crackers	Plantains	½ cup
Matzoh	¼ ounce	Potato (baked)	1-3 inch
Saltines	6 crackers	Potato (mashed)	½ cup
Wheat thins	8 crackers	Winter Squash	¾ cup
Popcorn (no fat added)	3 cups	Yam or sweet potato	½ cup (no sugar)

The Vegetable Group

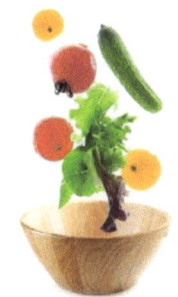

Any vegetable or 100 percent vegetable juice counts as a member of the Vegetable Group. Vegetables may be raw or cooked; fresh, frozen, canned, or dried/dehydrated. They also may be whole, cut-up, or mashed. Based on their nutrient content, vegetables are organized into 5 subgroups: dark green vegetables, starchy vegetables, red and orange vegetables, beans and peas, and other vegetables. The following table shows you food in each group and the suggested portion size. Remember butter, margarine, or fat (bacon fat) used to cook or top vegetables are counted as a fat serving.

THE VEGETABLE GROUP			
TYPE	COOKED	RAW	JUICE
Artichoke or artichoke hearts	½ cup	½ cup	
Asparagus	½ cup	½ cup	
Beans (green or yellow)	½ cup	½ cup	
Beets	½ cup	½ cup	
Broccoli	½ cup	½ cup	
Brussel sprouts	½ cup	½ cup	
Cabbage	no limit	no limit	
Carrots	½ cup	½ cup	½ cup
Cauliflower	½ cup	½ cup	
Celery	½ cup	½ cup	
Cucumber	½ cup	½ cup	
Eggplant	½ cup	½ cup	
Greens (collard, mustard, turnip)	½ cup	½ cup	
Kohlrabi	½ cup	½ cup	
Lettuce	no limit	no limit	
Miso	½ cup	½ cup	
Mixed vegetables (no corn or peas)	½ cup	½ cup	
Mushrooms	no limit	no limit	
Okra	½ cup	½ cup	
Onions	no limit	no limit	
Pea pods	½ cup	½ cup	
Peppers (green, red, yellow, or hot)	½ cup	½ cup	
Radishes	no limit	no limit	
Rutabaga	½ cup	½ cup	
Spinach	no limit	no limit	
Squash	½ cup	½ cup	
Tomato	½ cup	½ cup	½ cup
Turnips	½ cup	½ cup	
Water chesnuts	½ cup	½ cup	
Zucchini	no limit	no limit	

The Meat Group

Foods in this group include meats (like beef, chicken, and pork), fish (like salmon, tuna, and shrimp), meat substitutes (like tofu, and products that resemble meat or fish but are made with soy), eggs, and cheese. These foods are grouped together because the majority of the calories they contain come from protein and/or fat.

Cooked beans, peas, and lentils also are in this group because of the protein that they contain but are also considered starchy vegetables because of their carbohydrate content. While some meat substitutes and cheeses may contain small amounts of carbohydrate, the main macronutrients in these foods are protein and fat. Nuts are also often placed in this group because nuts contain some protein, but they are also high in fat.

Protein is very important in our daily diet. We need protein to maintain muscles, make enzymes, and keep our immune system working well. However, items in this group can be high in calories. Also, meat, eggs, and cheeses, in particular, can be high in saturated fat and cholesterol. People with diabetes need to make heart-healthy choices when choosing foods from this group because of their increased risk for cardiovascular complications.

Helpful Tips

- 1 serving = 1 ounce. A portion that fits in the palm of your hand = about 3 ounces or 3 servings.
- Coatings like flour or bread crumbs add carbohydrates and increase blood glucose.
- Bake, roast, broil, boil or grill meats instead of frying. Trim fat and skin. Use nonstick spray to cook.
- A serving of some fatty meats counts as a meat serving & fat serving. (See table)
- Canned meat, such as tuna, should be packed in water.

The following table shows food in each group and the suggested portion size.

THE MEAT GROUP

AMOUNT	TYPE	SERVING SIZE
1 OUNCE	Beef, Chicken, Turkey, Liver or Pork	1 slice (4" x 2" x ¼")
	Egg	1
	Cheese	1 ounce slice
	Cottage Cheese	1 cup
	Chicken	1 leg or wing
	Fish (Tuna, Salmon, Oysters, Shrimp, or Sardines)	¼ cup
	Lunchmeat	1 ounce slice
	Ground meat or stew meat	¼ cup
	Tempeh	¼ cup
	Peanut butter	2 tablespoons
2 OUNCE	Beef pattie	1 (2" x 2" x ½")
	Chicken thigh	1
	Chicken wings	2
	Egg with cheese	1 egg with 1 ounce of cheese
	Fish steak	1 (2" x 2" x ½")
	Meat tails or bones	½ cup
	Pork chop	1 small
	Tuna or Salmon (canned)	½ cup
3 OUNCE	Beef steak	1 (2" x 4" x ¾")
	Chicken	1 breast, 1 thigh or 2 drumsticks
	Egg omelet	2 eggs with 1 ounce of cheese
	Ground meat or stew meat	¾ cup cooked
	Meatballs	3
	Meatloaf	½ cup
	Pork Chop	1 medium
1 MEAT 1 FAT	Hot dog (polish kielbasa, country style)	1
	Sausage link	1 small
	Sausage pattie	1
	Smoked Sausage	1 ½

The Fats Group

Fat adds flavor to food and has little impact on your blood glucose, but is very high in calories and can lead to unwanted weight gain. Foods in this group include butter, margarine, salad dressing, mayonnaise, sour cream, oils, lard, and nuts. The foods in this group are grouped together because they contain similar amounts of calories and fat per serving and, with the exception of nuts, contain little protein or carbohydrates. Although fat is often thought of as being unhealthy for you, fat is essential for life. We need a certain amount of fat each day. The hard part is deciding what types and how much fat to eat.

There are four main types of fat, polyunsaturated, monounsaturated, trans, and saturated fats. All of these names describe the chemical structure of the different fats. Most foods contain a mixture of these four types of fats, but they are grouped by the type of fat that is present in the largest amount. While it is true that all fat is high in calories and that too much of any type of fat may be unhealthy, some types of fat are better for you than others. Saturated and trans fats have been shown to increase the risk for heart disease, but polyunsaturated and monounsaturated fats have been shown to have no effect on or decrease the risk for heart disease.

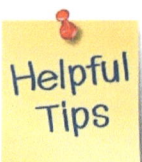

Tips for Choosing Foods from the Fats and Oils Group

- Choose foods that contain more polyunsaturated or monounsaturated fats rather than foods that contain saturated or trans fats.

- Choose low-fat or reduced-fat options when calories are similar to or less than the full-fat product. Sometimes the fat in low-fat products is replaced with carbohydrate, making a low-fat product that is still high in calories. For this reason, it is always important to check the calorie and macronutrient content of low-fat foods.
- Read the Nutrition Facts labels of foods to see how many grams of fat the products you consume contain.

The following table shows you food in each group and the suggested portion size.

The Fats Group

THE FATS GROUP		
	TYPE	**SERVING SIZE**
UNSATURATED FATS	Avocado	⅛ medium
	Margarine	1 teaspoon
	Margarine: Diet	1 tablespoon
	Mayonnaise	1 teaspoon
	Mayonnaise - *Reduced calorie*	1 tablespoon
	Miracle Whip	2 teaspoons
	Miracle Whip - *Reduced calorie*	1 tablespoon
	Olives - black	8 large
	Olives - green	10 large
	Salad dressing	1 tablespoon
	Salad dressing - *Reduced calorie*	2 tablespoons
	Tahini paste	2 teaspoons
	Oil *(Corn, Cotton seed, Safflower, Soybean, Sunflower, Olive & Peanut)*	1 teaspoon
	NUTS AND SEEDS	
	Almonds	8
	Cashews	5
	Pecans	5 halves
	Peanuts - small	20
	Peanuts - large	10
	Pistachios	1 ounce
	Pumpkin seeds	2 tablespoons
	Sunflower seeds	1 tablespoon
	Walnuts	5 halves
	Other nuts	1 tablespoon
SATURATED FATS	**SATURATED FATS**	
	Bacon	1 slice
	Bacon grease	1 teaspoon
	Butter	1 teaspoon
	Chitterlings	2 tablespoons
	Coconut - shredded	2 tablespoons
	Coffee creamer	1 tablespoon
	Cream cheese	1 tablespoon
	Cream cheese - reduced fat	1.5 tablespoons
	Cream - heavy	2 tablespoons
	Cream - light	2 tablespoons
	Lard	¼ ounce
	Shortening	1 teaspoon
	Sour cream	2 tablespoons

The Free Foods Group

Almost all foods contain calories, but some foods have so few that they aren't worth really counting. These are frequently called "free foods." A free food contains less than 20 calories per serving and can be used throughout the day for hunger.

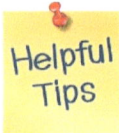

Helpful Tips

- Salt should be used in small amounts because it makes your body retain water which increases even normal swelling and may make your blood pressure higher. Use plenty of other herbs and seasonings that are salt-free.

- Caffeine is found primarily in coffee, tea, and soft drinks and should be limited while pregnant. You may have caffeinated drinks in small amounts (2 servings per day). Coffee and tea should be sweetened with sugar substitutes and whitened with milk instead of creamers.

The following table lists food in each group and the suggested portion size.

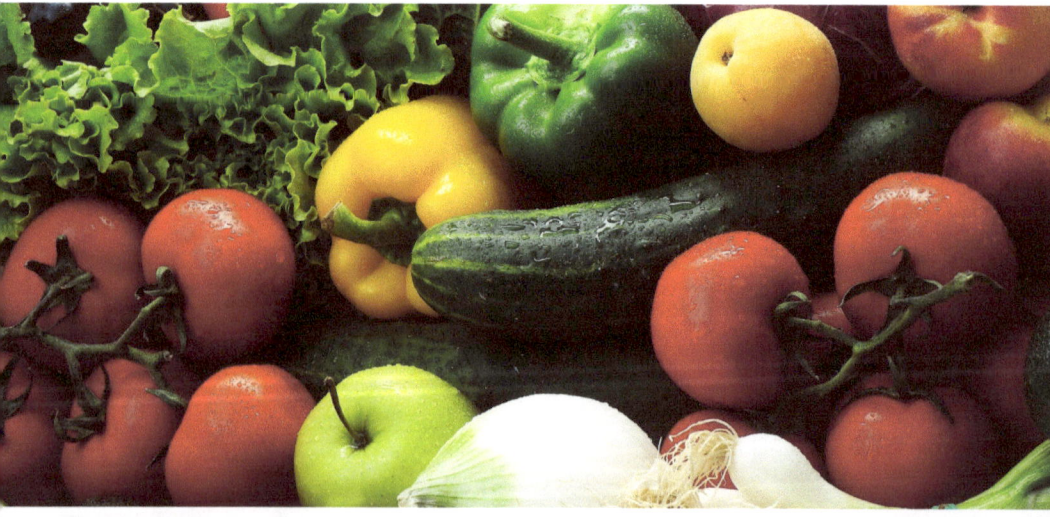

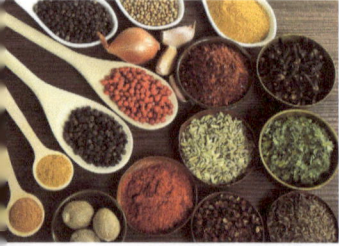
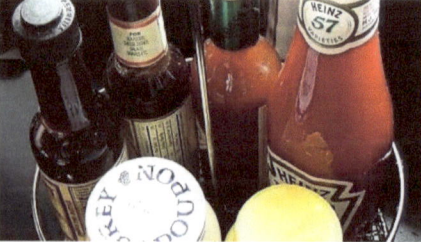
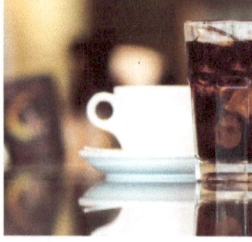

The Free Foods Group

THE FREE FOODS GROUP	
DRINKS	**VEGETABLES (RAW)**
Club Soda	Cabbage
Cocoa powder	Celery
Coffee	Cucumber
Drink mixes - (sugar free)	Lettuce - (Iceberg, Endive, Escarole, Romaine)
Soft drinks - (sugar free)	Mushrooms
Tea - (sugar free)	Onions - (green)
Water	Peppers - (hot)
Sugar Substitutes (Splenda, Truvia, Sweet'n'Low, Equal)	Radishes
	Zucchini
CONDIMENTS	
Coffee creamers - (nondairy powder)	Salad dressings
Cooking spray - (non-stick)	Salsa
Hot Sauce	Sour Cream
Jelly or Jam - (sugar free)	Soy Sauce
Lemon Juice	Syrup - (sugar free)
Mayonnaise or Miracle Whip	Vinegar
Mustard	Whipped Topping - (sugar free)
Reilish	Worcestershire Sauce
SNACKS	
Bouillon soup *(note: high in salt)*	Jell-O (sugar free)
Dill pickles	Popsicles (sugar free)
SPICES	
Basil	Oregano
Celery Seed	Paprika
Cinnamon	Pepper
Cumin	Pimento
Garlic powder	Salts - *(use in moderation)*
Onion powder	

Combination Foods

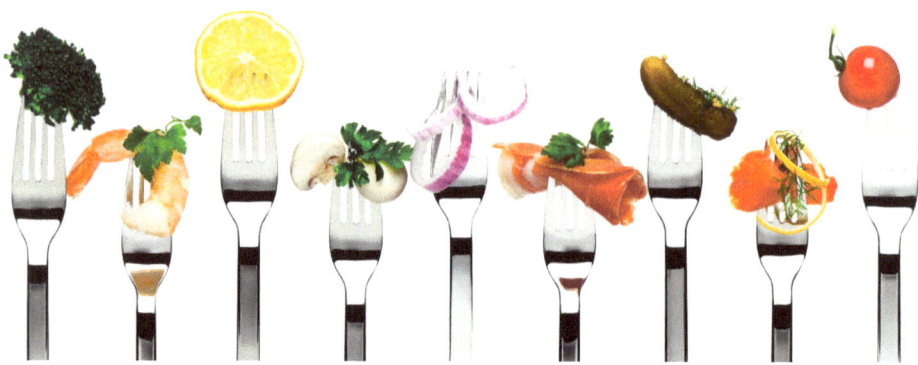

Combination foods are foods from different food categories that are eaten together. Eating combination foods means that the servings from each food category used must be counted.

- Remember to make all soups with water.
- Canned soups are very high is sodium (salt), and should be avoided.

	THE COMBINATION FOODS GROUP		
	FOOD TYPE	**SERVING SIZE**	**EXCHANGES PER SERVING**
SOUPS	Bean	1 cup	1 Carbohydrate & 1 Meat
	Chicken Noodle	1 cup	1 Carbohydrate & 1 Meat
	Cream	1 cup	1 Carbohydrate & 1 Fat
	Split pea	½ cup	1 Carbohydrate
	Tomato	1 cup	1 Carbohydrate
	Vegetable beef	1 cup	1 Carbohydrate
ENTREES	Casseroles - (Lasagna or Tuna)	1 cup	2 Carbs, 2 Meats, 1 Fat
	Chilli with beans	1 cup	2 Carbs, 2 Meats, 1 Fat
	Chow Mein	1 cup	1 Carb, 2 Meats, 2 Vegetables
	Macaroni and cheese	1 cup	2 Carbs, 1 Meat, 1 Fat
	Pizza - (thin crust with cheese)	¼ of 10 inch pizza	2 Carbs, 1 Meat, 1 Fat
	Pizza - (thin crust with meat)	¼ of 10 inch pizza	2 Carbs, 2 meats, 2 Fats
	Pot Pie	1-7 ounces	2 Carbs, 1 Meat, 4 Fats
	Spaghetti with meatballs	1 cup	2 Carbs, 2 Meats, 1 Fat

Combination Foods

Fast foods are quick and easy, however, they can also be high in carbohydrates, fat, salt, and calories. So it is important to carefully pay attention to portion sizes when eating fast foods. The following table lists samples of fast food menu options and suggested portion size.

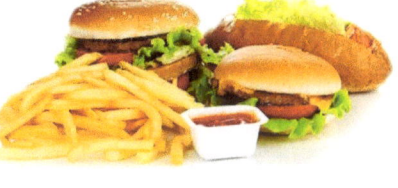

FAST FOODS		
FOOD TYPE B = Breakfast L/D=Lunch or Dinner	**SERVING SIZE**	**FOOD GROUPS PER SERVING**
B - McMuffin (Egg)	1	2 Carbs, 2 Meats, 1 Fat
B - McMuffin (Sausage)	1	2 Carbs, 1½ Meats, 2 Fats
B - Hashbrown	1	1 Carb, 1 Fat
L/D - Big Mac	1	3 Carbs, 2½ Meats, 3 Fats
L/D - Cheese Burger	1	2 Carbs, 2 Meats, 1 Fat
L/D - French Fries	Small	2 Carbs, 2 Fats
L/D - Hamburger	1	2 Carbs, 2 Meats, 1 Fat
L/D - Quarter Pounder w/Cheese	1	2 Carbs, 3½ Meats, 2 Fats
L/D - Salad (Chef)	1	2 Meats, 1 Vegetable
L/D - Salad (Chicken)	1	3 Meats, 1 Vegetable
L/D - Salad (Side)	1	1 Vegetable
L/D - Light Vinegrette	1 packet	1 Fat
L/D - Croutons	4 ounce pkg	½ Carbohydrate
L/D - Sub Sandwich w/ meat	6 inch	3 Carbs, 2 Meats, 2 Fats
Burrito - (Bean)	1	3½ Carbs, 1 Fat
Burrito - (Beef)	1	2½ Carbs, 2 Meats, 1 Fat
Burrito - (Chicken)	1	2½ Carbs, 2 Meats
Burrito - (Supreme)	1	3 Carbs, 1½ Meats, 2 Fats
Enchirito	1	2 Carbs, 2 Meats, 2 Fats
Gordita	1	2 Carbs, 2 Meats
Taco	1	1 Carb, 2 Meats
Tostada	1	2 Carbs, 1 Meat, 1 Fat

Foods to Avoid

Foods that have high amounts of simple sugar should be avoided until after the birth of your baby. These types of foods can make your blood glucose level very high. Once your baby is born, you may start to include small portions of the foods into your diet again.

FOODS TO AVOID
FOOD TYPE
Alcohol - (Beer, Liquor, Wine)
Bakery snacks - (i.e. Brownies, Twinkies, etc.)
Beverages - (i.e. Sugared Sodas, Kool-Aid, Sweet Tea)
Cakes
Candy
Cereal - (Sugar coated)
Chewing gum - (with sugar)
Coffee Lighteners - (i.e. Flavored creams, Coffee mate)
Cookies
Doughnuts
Frosting & Glazes
Honey
Ice Cream
Ice Milk
Jam
Jelly
Marmalade
Pastries
Pies
Sherbert
Sugar - (white granulated, brown)
Sweet Rolls
Syrup

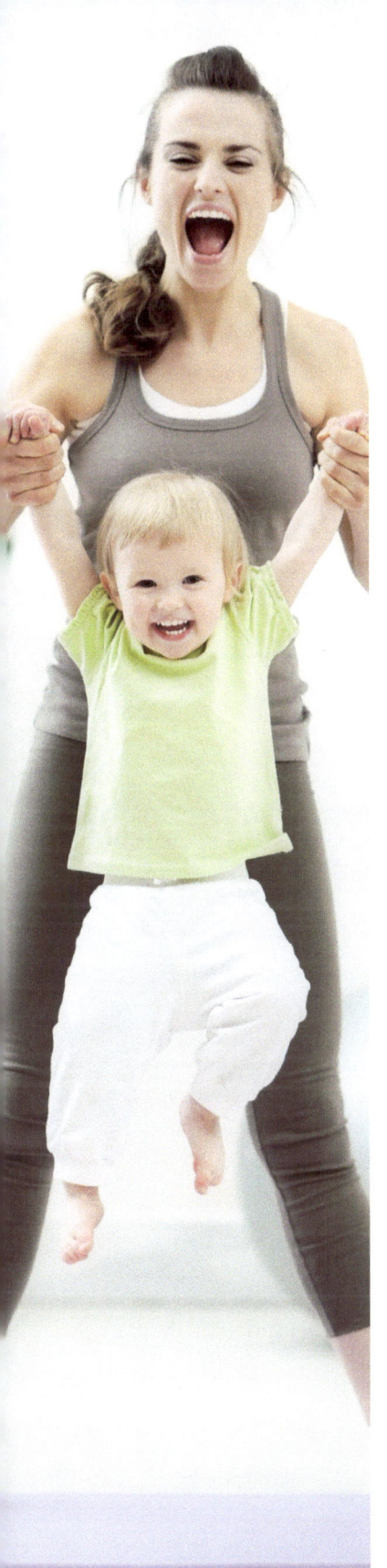

CHAPTER 4

STAYING HEALTHY AFTER PREGNANCY

After the Birth of Your Baby

Your health care provider will check your blood sugar level often, starting right after your baby is born. For most women, blood sugar levels go back to normal quickly after having their babies.

To ensure that diabetes has resolved it is very important to have a repeat Glucose Tolerance Test (GTT) at your 6-week postpartum visit. This test is similar to the one you took to find out whether or not you had gestational diabetes and based on the results of the test, you will fall into one of the following three categories:

AFTER PREGNANCY TEST CATEGORIES	
If your category is...	You should...
Normal	Get checked for diabetes every three years
Impaired Glucose Tolerance	Get checked for diabetes every year. Talk to your healthcare provider about ways to lower your risk level for diabetes.
Diabetic	Work with your healthcare provider to set up a treatment plan for your diabetes

The test also checks your risk for having diabetes in the future. About half of all women who have gestational diabetes are diagnosed with Type 2 Diabetes later in life.

Getting checked for diabetes is important because Type 2 Diabetes shows few symptoms. The only way to know for sure that you have Type 2 Diabetes is to have a blood test that reveals a higher than normal blood glucose level. You should also tell your healthcare provider right away if you notice any of the following:

- Being very thirsty
- Urinating often
- Feeling constantly or overly tired
- Losing weight quickly and/or without reason

Having one or more of these symptoms does not necessarily mean you have diabetes, but your health care provider might want to test you to make sure. Detecting Type 2 Diabetes early can help you avoid problems, like early heart disease and damage to your eyes, kidneys, or nerves. After pregnancy and in the future:

- Eat healthy foods and exercise regularly
- Have regular checkups
- Talk with your doctor about your plans for more children before your next pregnancy
- Watch your weight
- Plan to lose weight slowly. This will help you keep it off.

Eating healthy, maintaining weight in a healthy range and exercising regularly can help you delay or prevent Type 2 Diabetes in the future.

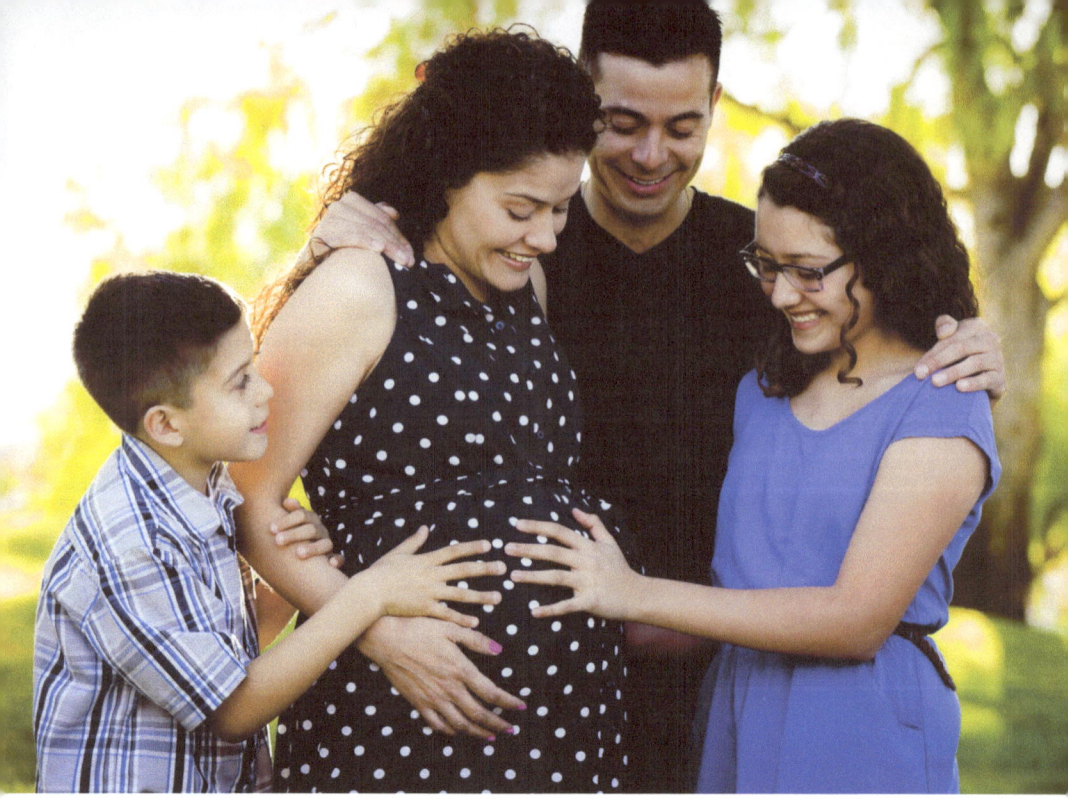

Future Pregnancies

Having developed diabetes during your pregnancy it is quite likely that it will reoccur in future pregnancies. Maintaining an ideal weight can help prevent this or help to control it if you do develop Gestational Diabetes.

If you know that you want to get pregnant in the future, have a blood sugar test up to three months before becoming pregnant to make sure you have a normal blood sugar level. If your blood sugar level is high, you may have developed Type 2 Diabetes without knowing it. As mentioned earlier in this booklet, high blood sugar early in the pregnancy (within the first eight weeks) can impact the developing body and organ systems of the fetus. So, it's important to get your blood sugar level under control before you get pregnant.

If you do get pregnant again, make sure your health care provider knows that you had Gestational Diabetes with your last pregnancy. If you had Gestational Diabetes with one pregnancy, your risk of getting it with another pregnancy is about 36 percent.

It may seem like a lot of work, but most women can successfully control their Gestational Diabetes and have healthy pregnancies. You can do it, too! Follow the treatment plan your health care provider designs for you.

A healthy pregnancy and a healthy birth are the greatest rewards.

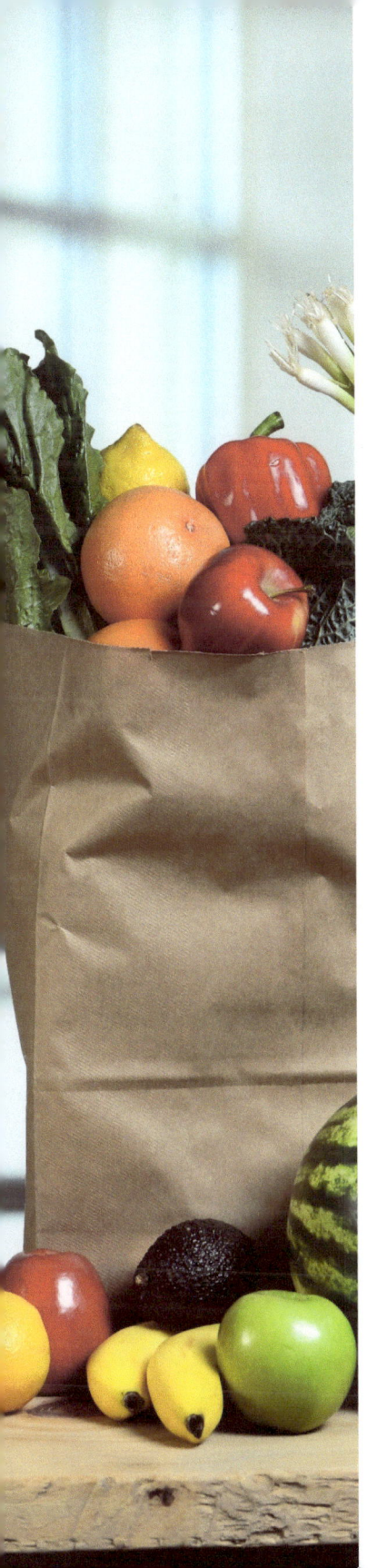

APPENDIX:
SAMPLE MENUS

Option 1

① Check your blood sugar (before eating breakfast)
Blood sugar goal 80-120mg/dl

② BREAKFAST

FOOD GROUP	MENU IDEAS	SERVING SIZE
Milk	1 cup milk	1
Fruit	Do not eat fruit for breakfast	0
Starch/Bread	1 slice of toast	1
Meat	1 egg	1
Fat	1 teaspoon butter	1

③ Check your blood sugar
(2 hours after eating breakfast)

*Blood Sugar Goal
80-120mg/dl*

④ MORNING SNACK

FOOD GROUP	MENU IDEAS	SERVING SIZE
Starch/Bread	¾ graham cracker	1
Meat	1 ounce cheese	1

⑤ LUNCH

FOOD GROUP	MENU IDEAS	SERVING SIZE
Milk	1 6oz light yogurt	1
Vegetables	Lettuce, tomato	2+
Fruit	1 small apple	1
Starch/Bread	1 hamburger bun	1
Meat	1 hamburger patty	2
Fat	1 tsp mayonnaise	1

⑥ Check your blood sugar
(2 hours after eating lunch)

*Blood Sugar Goal
80-120mg/dl*

⑦ AFTERNOON SNACK

FOOD GROUP	MENU IDEAS	SERVING SIZE
Starch/Bread	6 saltine crackers	1
Meat	1 ounce cheese	1

⑧ DINNER

FOOD GROUP	MENU IDEAS	SERVING SIZE
Milk	No milk servings	0
Vegetable	1 cup green beans	2+
Fruit	1 small apple	1
Starch/Bread	½ cup rice and corn	2
Meat	1 chicken breast	3
Fat	2 tsp butter	2

⑨ Check your blood sugar
(2 hours after eating lunch

*Blood Sugar Goal
80-120mg/dl*

⑩ BEDTIME SNACK

FOOD GROUP	MENU IDEAS	SERVING SIZE
Starch/Bread	3 cups popcorn	1
Meat	1 ounce cheese	1
Milk	½ cup pudding	1

Option 2

 Check your blood sugar (before eating breakfast)
Blood sugar goal 80-120mg/dl

 ## BREAKFAST

FOOD GROUP	MENU IDEAS	SERVING SIZE
Milk	1 cup milk	1
Fruit	Do not eat fruit for breakfast	0
Starch/Bread	½ cup cereal	1
Meat	1 sausage patty	1
Fat		0

 Check your blood sugar
(2 hours after eating breakfast)

*Blood Sugar Goal
80-120mg/dl*

 ## MORNING SNACK

FOOD GROUP	MENU IDEAS	SERVING SIZE
Starch/Bread	¾ graham cracker	1
Meat	2 tbsp peanut butter	1

 ## LUNCH

FOOD GROUP	MENU IDEAS	SERVING SIZE
Milk	1 cup milk	1
Vegetables	Grilled onions	2+
Fruit	1 small mango	1
Starch/Bread	2 tortillas	2
Meat	2 ounces of beef	2
Fat	⅛ of an avocado	1

 Check your blood sugar
(2 hours after eating lunch)

*Blood Sugar Goal
80-120mg/dl*

 ## AFTERNOON SNACK

FOOD GROUP	MENU IDEAS	SERVING SIZE
Starch/Bread	14 pretzels	2
Meat	2 Tbsp peanutbutter	1

 Check your blood sugar
(2 hours after eating lunch

*Blood Sugar Goal
80-120mg/dl*

DINNER

FOOD GROUP	MENU IDEAS	SERVING SIZE
Milk	No milk servings	0
Vegetable	Side Salad	1
Fruit	¼ cup pineapple	1
Starch/Bread	1 cup rice and beans	2
Meat	3 ounces chicken	3
Fat	1 Tbsp dressing	2

 ## BEDTIME SNACK

FOOD GROUP	MENU IDEAS	SERVING SIZE
Starch/Bread	1 slice bread	1
Meat	¼ cup chicken salad	1
Milk	1-6oz yogurt (light)	1

Check your blood sugar (before eating breakfast)
Blood sugar goal 80-120mg/dl

② BREAKFAST

FOOD GROUP	MENU IDEAS	SERVING SIZE
Milk	1 cup milk	1
Fruit	Do not eat fruit for breakfast	0
Starch/Bread	1 slice of toast	1
Meat	1 ounce cheese	1
Fat	1 tsp butter	1

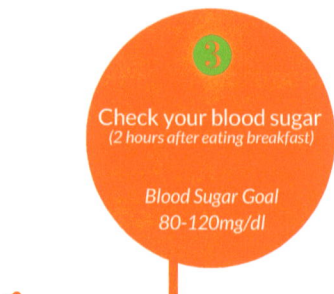

③ Check your blood sugar
(2 hours after eating breakfast)

*Blood Sugar Goal
80-120mg/dl*

④ MORNING SNACK

FOOD GROUP	MENU IDEAS	SERVING SIZE
Starch/Bread	½ bagel	1
Meat	2 Tbsp peanut butter	1

⑤ LUNCH

FOOD GROUP	MENU IDEAS	SERVING SIZE
Milk	1 cup milk	1
Vegetables	1 cup raw carrots	2+
Fruit	½ banana	1
Starch/Bread	2 slices bread	2
Meat	2 slices turkey	2
Fat	1 tsp mayonnaise	1

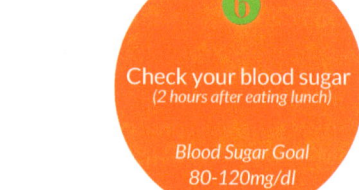

⑥ Check your blood sugar
(2 hours after eating lunch)

*Blood Sugar Goal
80-120mg/dl*

⑦ AFTERNOON SNACK

FOOD GROUP	MENU IDEAS	SERVING SIZE
Starch/Bread	14 pretzels	2
Meat	1 ounce cheese	1

⑧ DINNER

FOOD GROUP	MENU IDEAS	SERVING SIZE
Milk	No milk servings	0
Vegetable	1 small apple	1
Fruit	1 cup green beans	1
Starch/Bread	½ cup rice and corn	2
Meat	1 chicken breast	3
Fat	2 tsp butter	2

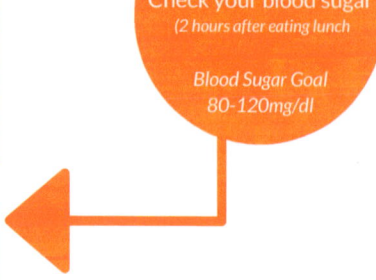

⑨ Check your blood sugar
(2 hours after eating lunch)

*Blood Sugar Goal
80-120mg/dl*

⑩ BEDTIME SNACK

FOOD GROUP	MENU IDEAS	SERVING SIZE
Starch/Bread	1 slice bread	1
Meat	¼ cup chicken salad	1
Milk	1-6oz yogurt (light)	1

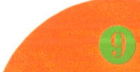

Sample Blood Glucose Log

Date	Breakfast		Lunch		Dinner		Insulin/ Medication	Notes
	Before	After	Before	After	Before	After		

REFERENCES

Allender, J., Rector, C. & Warner, K. (2010). Community Health Nursing: Promoting & protecting the public's health (7th ed.). Philadelphia: Wolters Kluwer / Lippincott Williams & Wilkins.

American College of Obstetricians and Gynecologists Practice Bulletin: Clinical management guidelines for obstetricians-gynecologists. Number 137, August 2013. Obstetrics and Gynecology 122(2):406, 2013.

American Diabetes Association. Classification and diagnosis of diabetes. Sec. 2. In Standards of Medical Care in Diabetes -2017. Diabetes Care 2017;40(Suppl. 1):S11–S24.

American Diabetes Association: Gestational Diabetes Mellitus (Position Statement). Diabetes Care 26(Suppl 1): S103-S105, 2003. Metzger BE, Coustan DR (Eds.): Proceedings of the Fourth International Workshop Conference on Gestational Diabetes Mellitus. Diabetes Care 21(Suppl. 2): B1-B167, 1998.

American Diabetes Association. Glycemic targets. Sec. 6. In Standards of Medical Care in Diabetesd2017. Diabetes Care 2017;40(Suppl. 1):S48–S56.

American Diabetes Association. Lifestyle management. Sec. 4. In Standards of Medical Care in Diabetesd2017. Diabetes Care 2017;40(Suppl. 1):S33–S43.

Barnes-Powel, L. (2007). Infants of diabetic mothers: The effects of hyperglycemia on the fetus and neonate. Neonatal Network 26 (5).

Begley, A. (2002). Barriers to good nutrient intakes during pregnancy: A qualitative analysis. Nutrition & Dietetics 59 (3).

Berzin, R., Hulbert, D.(2001). My doctor says I have gestational diabetes…what do I do now? Becton Dickinson Consumer Products.

Buchanan, T., Xiang, A., Kjos, S. & Watanabe, R. (2006). What is gestational diabetes? American Diabetes Association.

Centers for Disease Control and Prevention. National Diabetes Fact Sheet: National Estimates and General Information on Diabetes and Prediabetes in the United States, 2011. .s.l. : U.S. Department of Health and Human Services, Centers for Disease Control and Prevention, 2011

Chung, J.H., Voss,, K.J., Caughey, A.B., Wing, D.A., Henderson, E.J. & Major, C.A., (2006). Role of patient education level in predicting macrosomia among women with gestation diabetes mellitus. Journal of Perinatology 26, 328-332, doi:10.1038/sj.jp.7211512.

Cloherty, J., Eichenwald, E., Stark, A. (2008). Manual of neonatal care 6th ed. Philadelphia: Lippincott Williams & Wilkins.

Cordero, L., Treuer, S., Landon, M., Gabbe, S. (1998). Management of infants of diabetic mothers. Archives Pediatric Adolescent Medicine 152.

Dossey, B., Keegan, L., & Guzzetta, C. (2005). Pocket guide for holistic nursing. Boston: Jones and Bartlett.

Edelman, C. & Mandle, C. (2010). Health promotion throughout the lifespan (7th ed.). Canada: Mosby / Elsevier.

Funnell, M., Brown, T., Childs, B., Haas, L., Hosey, G., Jensen, B…Weis, M. (2006). National standards for diabetes self-management education. American Diabetes Association.

Garcia-Patterson, A., Martin, E., Ubeda, J., Maria, M., Adelantado, J., Ginovart, G., Corcoy, R. (2002). Nurse-base management in patients with gestational diabetes-Diabetes Care. American Diabetes Association. Retrieved from http://care.diabetesjournals.org/content/26/4/998.full.

Gonder-Frederic, L., Cox, D., & Ritterband, L. (2002). Diabetes and behavioral medicine: The second decade. Journal of Counseling and Clinical Psychology, 70(3), 611-625. doi:10.1037//0022-006X.70.3.611.

Jobson Medical (2011). Medication compliance in diabetes: A strategic guide for the practicing pharmacist. Retrieved from http://www.powerpak.com/index.aspshow=lesson&page=courses/2995/lesson.htm&lsn_id=2995.

Jovanovic, L. (2007). Diabetes in pregnancy. Retrieved from http://www.presentdiabetes.com/lecture_hall/description.php?id=254.

Keohane, N., Lacey, L. (May/June 1991). Preparing the woman with gestational diabetes for self-care. Journal of Obstetric, Gynecologic & Neonatal Nursing. Retrieved from http://onlinelibrary.wiley.com/doi/10.1111/j.1552-6909.1991.tb02530.x/pdf.

Mensing, C. & Norris, S. (2003). Group education in diabetes: Effectives and implementation. Diabetes Spectrum 16 (2).

Norris SL, Lau J, Smith SJ, Schmid CH, Engelgau MM. Self-management education for adults with type 2 diabetes: a meta-analysis of the effect on glycemic control. s.l. : Diabetes Care, 2002. pp. 25:1159– 1171

Renshaw, R. (2007). Keys to Diabetes Control? Patience, Persistence, and Perseverance. MANAGED CARE. Retrieved from https://www.managedcaremag.com/archives/2007/5/keys-diabetes-control-patience-persistence-and-perseverance.

Roche Diagnostics (2010). Acch-check Aviva meter system. Operator's manual. Retrieved February 13, 2011 from https://www.accu-chek.com/us/glucose-meters/aviva-how-to-use.html.

Schumacher, E. (2005). Diabetes self-management: Education: the key to living well with diabetes. Retrieved from http://www.dcmsonline.org/jax-medicine/2005journals/diabetes/diab05j-pt-education.pdf.

Spikmans, F.J.M., Brugg, J., M.M.B. Doven, Kruizenda, H.M., Hofsteenge, G. H., &Van-Bokhurst-van der Schueren, M.A.E. (2003). Why do diabetic patients not attend appointments with their dietician? Journal of Human Nutrition and Dietetics 16. Retrieved from http://onlinelibrary.wiley.com/doi/10.1046/j.1365-277X.2003.00435.x/abstract.

Thomas, A & Gutierrez, Y. (2005). American Dietetic Association guide to gestational diabetes mellitus. USA.

Tieu J., Crowther C.A., & Middleton P. (2008). Dietary advice in pregnancy for preventing gestational diabetes mellitus. The Cochrane Collaboration. Retrieved from http://www.cfah.org/hbns/archives/viewSupportDoc.cfm?supportingDocID=588.

Verklan, M. & Ealden, M. (2004). Core curriculum for neonatal intensive care nursing 3rd ed. USA: Elsevier Saunders.